I0436380

Cyclist's Notebook: For ideas, thoughts, projects, plans, lists and notes.

Dubreck World Publishing

Copyright

'Cyclist's Notebook: For ideas, thoughts, projects, plans, lists and notes.'

First published in July 2021 by Dubreck World Publishing
Printed and bound by Lulu Press
Distributed by Lulu Press

ISBN-13: 978-1-326-52122-6
First Edition

DUBRECK WORLD PUBLISHING

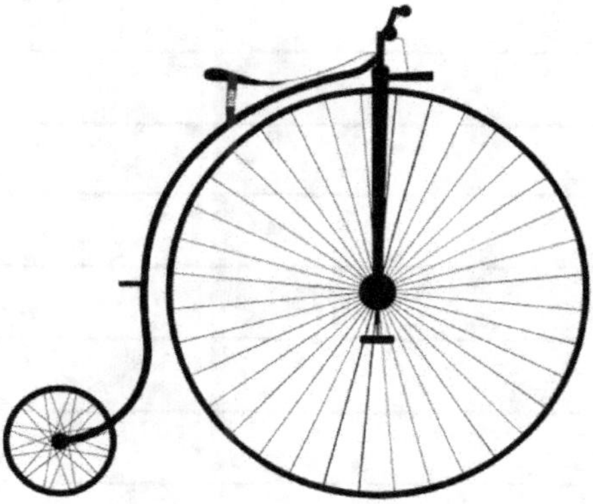

This book belongs to

……………………………………………………………………………………………

www.ingramcontent.com/pod-product-compliance
Lightning Source LLC
Chambersburg PA
CBHW060109300526
45791CB00018B/878
* 9 7 8 1 3 2 6 5 2 1 2 2 6 *